HOW TO LIVE a HEALTHY LIVE

TAOSIFAT OLADEJO

TABLE OF CONTENTS

NUTRITION

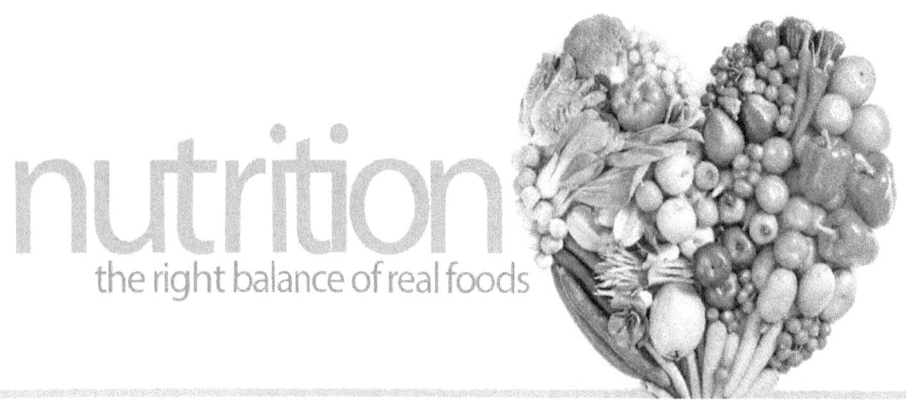

Nutrition is about eating a healthy and balanced diet. Food and drink provide the energy and nutrients you need to be healthy. Understanding these nutrition terms may make it easier for you to make better food choices.

You need to eat nutritious meals to be healthy. This is because eating nutritious meals will help you grow up and do well in every activities. When you eat nutritious food, you'll be full of energy and you will not fall sick easily.

What is a nutritious meal?

A nutritious meal is a meal that has the six classes of food served in the right amounts. All the six classes of food may not be contained in a single meal. However it is encouraged to take meals that contain these six classes in a day.

The classes of food are:

Carbohydrates	Bread, Rice, Maize etc
Protein	Meat, Fish, Eggs etc
Fats and Oil	Butter, Olive oil etc
Minerals	Nuts and seeds, Shellfish
Vitamins	Fruits and vegetables
Water	H20

These nutrient classes can be categorized as either macronutrients (needed in relatively large amounts) or micronutrients (needed in smaller quantities). The macronutrients are carbohydrates, fats, fiber, proteins, and water. The micronutrients are minerals and vitamins.

Carbohydrates are one of the most consumed class of food. Carbohydrates contain a lot of starch and supply glucose to the human body, which the body transforms into energy to help the body function efficiently. Carbohydrate-rich foods are an important part of a balanced diet.

Sources of Carbohydrates: The healthiest carbohydrate sources are unprocessed or slightly processed whole grains, vegetables, fruits, and legumes, which provide vitamins, minerals, fiber, and a variety of phytonutrients.

White bread, pastries, sodas, and other highly processed or refined meals are all unhealthy sources of carbs. These foods are high in easily digestible carbohydrates, which can cause weight gain, obstruct weight loss, and promote diabetes and heart disease.

Protein's importance can be seen in the muscle-building process, in the transmission of messages, and in hair growth. Protein is high in energy; this energy can be obtained from the meat we eat, and this meat provides additional resources for the development of complex nervous systems and a healthy brain.

A high-protein diet is essential for children, pregnant and nursing women, and those healing from an accident because of this energy.

Sources of Proteins: There are also ten important proteins that humans require but cannot produce on their own. That means the only way we can receive these essential proteins is through our diet. Beans, meat, dairy, eggs, whole grains, soy products, and legumes are good sources of protein foods.

Fats are a great source of energy. Approximately no more than 35% of our daily calories should come from fat.

Fat protects internal organs, but too much of it might be harmful. Fat is also a good insulator, and fat stored just beneath the skin helps to keep the body warm. Because fat cells secrete and store oestrogen, females need a certain amount of body fat to sustain menstruation function.

Fat and oil are generally portrayed and categorized as a single entity. Fats are fatty compounds that are solid or semi-solid triglycerides, whereas oils are transparent liquids.

Minerals are natural elements that can be found in the soil. Plants absorb them, and we consume them, or animals eat them, and we eat them. As a result, minerals can be obtained from both animal and vegetable sources.

Minerals play a variety of tasks, from structural to regulatory, such as calcium in bones and teeth and sodium and potassium in fluid balance and muscle contractions.

Minerals include calcium and iron amongst many others found in meat, cereals, fish, dairy foods, fruit & vegetables, and nuts.

Vitamins are complex organic molecules contained in food that supports nearly every human system, including the immune system, brain, and neurological system. Many of them aid in the conversion of food into energy and the utilization of glucose, fat, and protein by the body.

Vitamins A, C, B6, and D are among the 13 essential vitamins that the body requires to function properly. Vitamins are necessary for clear vision, healthy skin, and strong bones. Eat foods that are as fresh and unprocessed as possible to acquire extra vitamins in your diet.

Water, along with carbs, proteins, and lipids, is one of the most significant macronutrients. We can survive without food for a little longer (about 8 weeks) than we can without water (only a few days).

Our bodies are made up of about 65 percent water, which helps with absorption, digestion, excretion, and nutrient circulation.

Lack of fluids may cause you to become tired, making fixation and execution more difficult. It plays a larger role in the body's absorption, body temperature regulation, reproduction, food transit, oxygen transport, and other chemical issues.

A healthy balanced diet includes all three macronutrients in moderation, plus a wide enough variety of foods to access all your required vitamins and minerals. In other words, nutrients are things that humans need to consume in order to survive and to thrive.

FOOD HYGIENE

Food Hygiene, otherwise known as Food Safety can be defined as handling, preparing and storing food or drink in a way that best reduces the risk of consumers becoming sick from the food-borne disease. The principles of food safety aim to prevent food from becoming contaminated and causing food poisoning.

Food hygiene is what you need to do to keep food clean from the time it is taken from the farm till it is prepared and eaten.

The key principles for safe food preparation are outlined below.

- Choose foods that are not easily damaged by transportation, accident or by storage.

- Cook foods thoroughly, especially meat because this can help to kill any microorganism that might be present in the food.
- Eat cooked foods immediately after they are cooked rather than leave them out and eat later.
- Store cooked food carefully at an appropriate temperature.
- If food must be reheated, be sure to reheat it thoroughly.
- Avoid contact between raw and cooked food.
- Wash hands properly before handling food and before eating.
- Keep all kitchen surfaces and utensils meticulously clean.
- Protect food from animals including insects, rodents and other animals.

- Use safe water in food preparation and for washing fruits and vegetables to be eaten raw.
- Cover food so that flies and dogs do not have contact with it.
- Stop food like rice and beans in clean, dry places where rats and cockroaches cannot get to.
- Wash all spoons and other things you use to cook food.

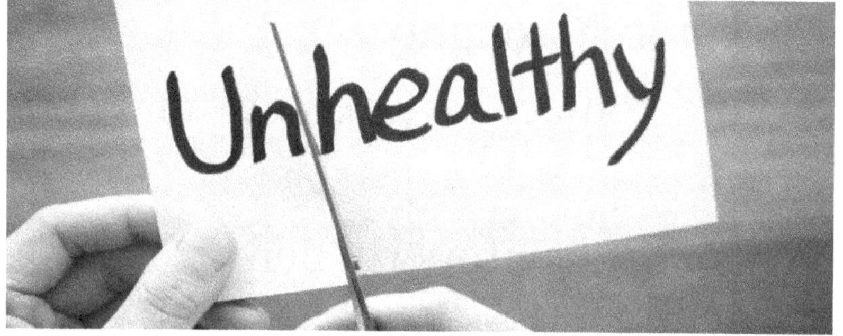

People who eat a lot of unhealthy and unhygienic food are more likely to develop heart diseases and other health problems. As we know, eating a healthy diet is very important for maintaining a healthy lifestyle.

PERSONAL AND ENVIRONMENTAL HYGIENE

To live and stay healthy, unique personnel and environmental hygiene.

What is personal and environmental hygiene?

This means keeping your body and the area where you live clean. Good personal hygiene involves keeping all parts of the external body clean and healthy. It is important for maintaining both physical and mental health.

You need to keep your body clean by:

- Taking a bath everyday with soap and clean water.
- Washing your hands with soap hard water before eating and after using the toilet.

- Washing your hands with soap and water once you get back into the house after returning from school or work.
- Washing your hands after playing or touching your pets like dogs or cats.
- Not sharing your underwear with anybody.
- Not sharing towels with anybody.
- Not sharing toothbrushes with anyone else.
- Brushing your teeth in the morning when you wake up and before going to bed.
- Keeping finger and toe nails shout and clean.
- Keeping your clothes clean by washing them regularly.
- Making your water clean enough to drink it either by boiling.

You need to keep your environment clean by:

- Sweeping and cleaning your house.
- Sweeping and cleaning the areas surrounding your house.
- Clearing gutters surrounding your house.
- Throwing away dirts into the dustbin and covering it after use.
- Sleeping away water that collects near your house.
- Cutting overgrown bushes anywhere near your house.

Keeping the body clean has positive effects on a person's social life and their physical and mental health. Personal hygiene is simply looking after the body and keeping it clean and healthy. Developing and maintaining a personal hygiene routine is key to having a healthy body and mind.

EXERCISE

What is exercise?

This simply means being active. In simple terms, exercise is any movement that works your body at a greater intensity than your usual level of daily activity. Exercise raises your heart rate and works your muscles and is most commonly undertaken to achieve the aim of physical fitness

Benefits of Exercise

- Exercise can make you happier.
- Exercise can help with weight loss.
- Exercise is good for your muscles and bones.
- Exercise can increase your energy levels.
- Exercise can reduce your risk of chronic disease.
- Exercise can help skin health.

- Exercise can help your brain health and memory.
- Exercise can help with relaxation and sleep quality.
- Exercise can reduce pain.
- Exercise helps you to digest food faster.
- Your body will be able to fight infections better.
- Your body releases chemicals called endorphins which makes you feel good.

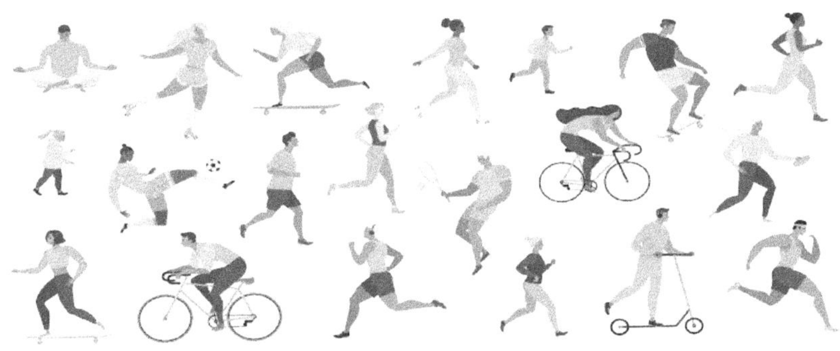

Exercise offers incredible benefits that can improve nearly every aspect of your health. Regular physical activity can increase the production of hormones that make you feel happier and help you sleep better.

What are the types of exercise?

- Climbing staircase
- Cycling
- Playing football
- Swinging
- Squats
- Push ups
- Jumping jacks
- Side planks
- Crunches etc

Exercise is the miracle cure we've always had, but for too long we've neglected to take our recommended dose. Our health is now suffering as a consequence.

People who exercise regularly have a lower risk of developing many long-term (chronic) conditions, such as heart disease, type 2 diabetes, stroke, and some cancers.

AVOIDING UNHEALTHY PRACTICES

To live and stay healthy, you must keep away from some things.

These includes;

- Smoking: Do not smoke. It increases your risk of getting lung cancer.
- Alcohol: Do not drink. It could make you misbehave and have accident that could be prevented. It increases the risk of having liver problems and other diseases.
- Do not take hard drugs like Indian hemp, cocaine, heroine, morphine etc. It could lead you into bad behavior and also cause mental problems.
- Do not share toothbrushes and towels. It could cause skin and mouth disease.
- Not getting enough sleep.

- Eating late at night.
- Be careful when using dangerous objects like knives and other sharp objects.
- Eating too much junk food.
- Not having enough exercise.
- Not drinking enough water.
- Eating an unhealthy diet.
- Not keeping the environment clean.

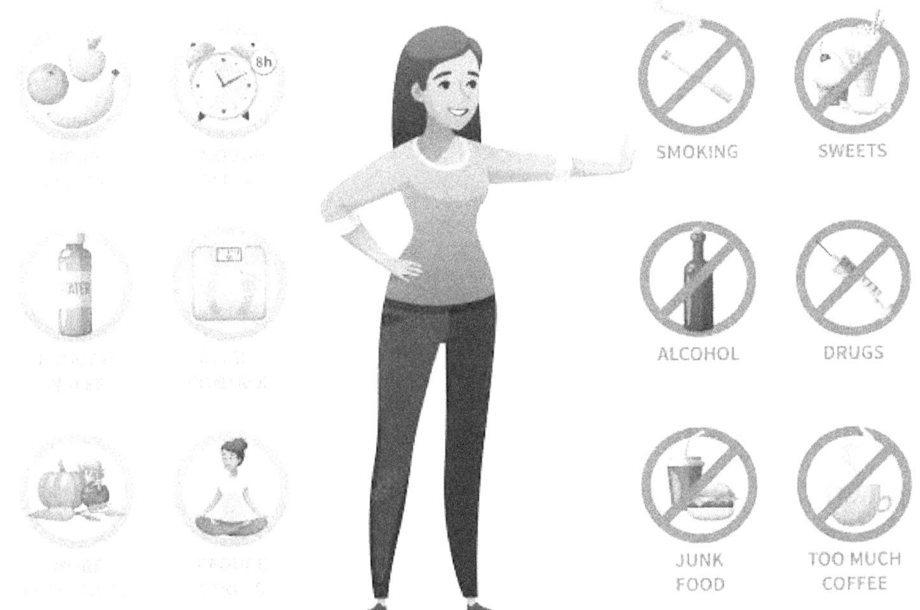

Millions of people follow an unhealthy lifestyle. Hence, they encounter illness, disability and even death.

Problems like metabolic diseases, joint and skeletal problems, cardio-vascular diseases, hypertension, overweight, violence and so on, can be caused by an unhealthy lifestyle.

Physical inactivity, along with increasing tobacco use and poor diet and nutrition, are increasingly becoming part of today's lifestyle leading to the rapid rise of diseases such as cardiovascular diseases, diabetes, or obesity.

Eating a healthy, balanced diet is an important part of maintaining good health, and can help us feel our best.
Keep yourself healthy!

PREVENTING DISEASE

Disease prevention is a procedure through which individuals, particularly those with risk factors for a disease, are treated in order to prevent a disease from occurring. Treatment normally begins either before signs and symptoms of the disease occur, or shortly thereafter.

Infectious diseases are caused by microscopic organisms that live in other people, animals, or the environment and are too small to see. While specific diseases are passed in specific ways, there are basic steps you can take to stay healthy and lower your risk of catching and spreading any infectious disease.

What you should do?

- Keep immunizations up to date.
- Use antibiotics exactly as prescribed.
- Report to your doctor any quickly worsening infection or any infection that does not get better after you take a prescribed antibiotic.
- If you travel internationally, get all recommended immunizations, and use protective medications for travel, especially to areas with malaria.

- Wash your hands often, especially during cold and flu season.
- Be aware of what you eat, and prepare foods carefully.
- Be cautious around all wild and domestic animals that are not familiar to you.
- After any animal bite, clean the skin with soap and water, and seek medical care immediately.
- Avoid areas where there are ticks.
- Protect yourself from mosquitoes.
- Stay alert to disease threats when you travel or visit undeveloped areas.
- Don’t drink untreated water while hiking or camping. If you become ill when you return home, tell your doctor where you’ve been.
- If you are sick with a cold or flu, stay home and don't spread germs.
- Practice safer sex.

- Do not use intravenous drugs or share syringes.
- Weigh your weight regularly and be cautious of being obese.

Chronic diseases are the leading causes of death and disability.

The good news is that you have the power to help prevent chronic disease, as making positive diet and lifestyle changes can help reduce risk. Eating healthy foods, getting enough exercise, and refraining from tobacco and excessive alcohol use confer numerous health benefits—including possibly preventing the onset of chronic diseases.

ABC OF HEALTHY LIVING

A; Avoid smoking.
Avoid drinking alcohol.
Avoid taking drugs without prescription.

Avoid fighting which can cause injuries.

B; Bath everyday

Brush your teeth in the morning and at night.

C; Cut your finger and toenails properly.

Clothes should be kept clean by washing and drying properly.

D; Diet, eat nutritious food.

Don't share toothbrushes and towels.

E; Exercise regularly.

Environment should be kept clean always.

OTHERS;

- Rest and sleep well every day.
- Wash your hands before you eat and after using the toilet.

- Follow and learn by heart all that you've read above.

CONCLUSION

Healthy living is having the opportunity, capability and motivation to act in a way that positively affects your physical and mental well-being. Paying attention to what you eat, being physically active, and learning more about your food and yourself can help you meet your health goals.

When you’re not at your healthiest, you can probably tell. You may simply feel “off.” You may find that you feel tired, your digestive system isn’t functioning as well as it normally does. Mentally, you may find out you can’t concentrate and feel anxious or depressed.

The good news: a healthy lifestyle can help you feel better. Even better, you don't have to overhaul your entire life overnight. It's pretty easy to make a couple of small changes that can steer you in the direction of improved well-being. And once you make one change, that success can motivate you to continue to make more positive shifts.

Ready to level up healthy living? Take that bold step today.

www.ingramcontent.com/pod-product-compliance
Lightning Source LLC
LaVergne TN
LVHW060839170826
845678LV00007B/1815

9798844201165